THE SKIN
Coverings and Linings
of Living Things

THE SKIN

COVERINGS AND LININGS
OF LIVING THINGS

Dr. Alvin Silverstein
and
Virginia B. Silverstein

Illustrated by Lee J. Ames

PRENTICE-HALL, INC., Englewood Cliffs, N.J.

For Sidney and Ruth Silvers

The authors would like to thank Dr. John Reeves of the United States Public Health Service for his valuable comments and suggestions.

THE SKIN: Coverings and Linings of Living Things
by Alvin Silverstein and Virginia B. Silverstein

Printed in the United States of America • J

Prentice-Hall International, Inc., London
Prentice-Hall of Australia, Pty. Ltd., North Sydney
Prentice-Hall of Canada, Ltd., Toronto
Prentice-Hall of India Private Ltd., New Delhi
Prentice-Hall of Japan, Inc., Tokyo

Library of Congress Cataloging in Publication Data

Silverstein, Alvin.
    THE SKIN: coverings and linings of living things.

    SUMMARY: Describes the composition and function of the human skin and the inner linings of the body as well as such animal coverings as feathers, furs, and scales.
    1. Skin—Juvenile literature. [1. Skin]
I. Silverstein, Virginia B., joint author. II. Ames, Lee J., illus. III. Title.
PZ10.S664Sk   612'.79   72-2004
ISBN 0-13-812776-X

10   9   8   7   6   5   4   3   2

CONTENTS

31985

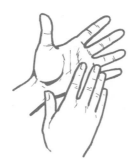

1

Coverings Outside and In

Look at the palm of your left hand. Run the fingertips of your right hand across it. It feels smooth, but it does not look smooth. There are many lines and creases in your palm, and they do not disappear even if you stretch your hand out.

What about the back of your hand? Do you see any differences? Do you see any tiny hairs? Look at the hard fingernails at the tips of your fingers.

Everything you have seen on your hand is skin, or things that the skin has made. Your whole body is covered with skin. This covering is as snug-fitting and flexible as a surgeon's fine rubber gloves. But it is far more complicated. Skin protects you from germs and from injury. It helps to cool you in the summertime and keep you warm in the winter. It helps to tell you about the world around you—the shapes and textures of things, and whether they

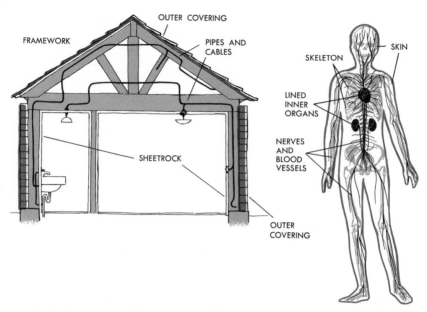

Both house and human have outer coverings and inner linings.

are hot or cold. The skin is a living covering that grows with you and repairs itself when it is damaged.

In some ways, your body is like the house you live in. A house has an outer covering of brick or stucco or shingles that protects it from the rain and wind. Inside the walls is a framework that supports the house, and various pipes and electric cables that carry water and electricity. The walls of the house have an inner covering, too, made of plaster or sheetrock, which may in turn be covered with wallpaper or paint.

The outer covering of your body is your skin. Your inner supporting framework is a skeleton made of bones. Blood vessels carry fluids and nerves carry messages to all parts of your body. The parts of your body—the blood vessels, nerves, and various organs such as the heart and kidneys— each have their own outer coverings. They are wrapped in a kind of tissue called *epithelial* (EP-IH-THEEL-EE-UL) tissue. The insides of these organs are lined with more epithelial tissue.

There are three main kinds of epithelial tissue in the body. The cells in the outer part of your skin belong to the type called *squamous* (SKWAH-MUSS) *epithelium*. The name "squamous" comes from a word meaning "scale." Under a microscope, squamous epithelium looks like an arrangement of scales or pavement stones. It is made of thin, flat cells that are joined together at the edges.

You can see some squamous epithelial cells for yourself, if you have a microscope. Using the flat edge of a toothpick, *gently* scrape the inside of your cheek. A tiny bit of epithelium will come off onto the toothpick. It may be so small that you may not even see it, yet this bit of material may contain hundreds or even thousands of squamous epithelial cells. Smear the material on a microscope slide and place a drop of iodine on it. Now look at it under a microscope. When you see the squamous epithelial cells under high power, you will notice that there is a dark spot near the center of each cell. This is the nucleus. You would not have been able to see the cells and their nuclei as well without the iodine, which colors them.

Squamous epithelial cells are also found in the inner walls of blood vessels and lining the inside of the lungs, kidneys, and other parts of the body.

A second type of epithelial tissue is made up of cells that look like tiny cubes. The type is called *cuboidal* (CUE-BOYD-AL) *epithelium*. It is found in many glands, such as the thyroid gland, in the lens of the eye, and in the kidneys.

By far the most common type of epithelium is *columnar epithelium.* You can guess from its name that it is made up of cells that look like little columns or fence posts. There are many different kinds of columnar epithelium. These long, slim cells, for example, line the stomach, intestines, and digestive glands. Some of the cells in these linings are special. They do not look exactly like columns; instead they look like a tiny goblet. These *goblet cells* produce or secrete enzymes that help digest the foods we eat.

A different kind of columnar epithelium lines the respiratory tract, from the nose down to the tiny branches in the lungs. These columnar cells are topped by a fringe of many hairlike structures called *cilia* (SILL-EE-UH). These cilia wave back and forth together in rhythm. They help to keep

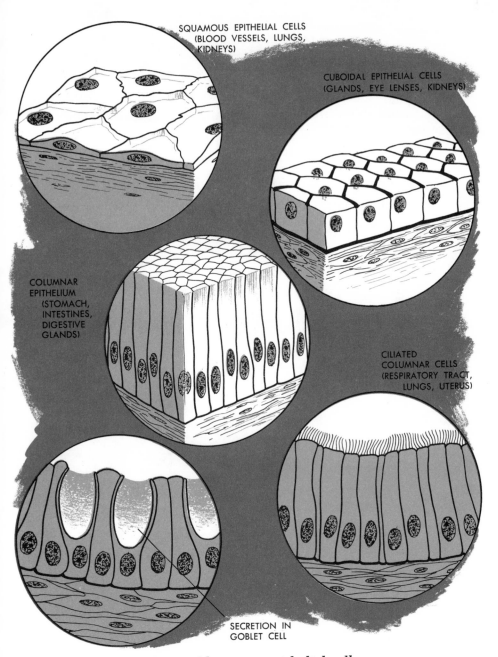

Types of lining or epithelial cells.

5

dust particles out of the lungs and move them upward so that they can be coughed or sneezed out.

Ciliated columnar epithelium is also found in the uterus and in tubes of the reproductive system in men and women.

Basically the same kinds of epithelial tissues are found in cats and dogs, elephants and fish, birds and snakes—in all the higher animals. Indeed, all living things, from fleas to trees, have covering tissues of one kind or another.

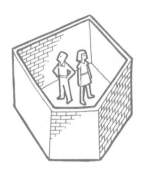

2

The Wall Around Us

Is your skin alive or dead? Alive, of course, you would say. Otherwise, how could it grow with you? But think for a moment. When you get a sunburn, flakes of skin peel off. This skin is not alive. Have you ever noticed bits of peeling skin coming off when you dry yourself after a bath?

You are actually losing skin cells all the time, even when you do not notice it. When you shake hands with a friend, you leave some of your skin cells with him. When you take your clothes off at night, and when you put your clothes on in the morning, skin cells are rubbed off your body. Every time you wash your hands, skin cells go down the drain.

You do not have to worry. The outer skin cells that you lose so easily are not alive. Indeed, the whole outer layer of your skin is made up of dead cells. They were once alive, a part of the living layer of the skin called the *epidermis* (EP-IH-*DER*-MISS*). But new living epidermal cells were formed beneath them, and new cells under them in turn. Gradually the older epidermal cells worked their way outward, toward the surface of the skin, as the outer dead cells were rubbed or flaked away. An average skin cell lives just 28 days.

What makes the outer cells of the epidermis die? The tiny blood vessels that nourish the skin cells are found just under the bottom of the epidermis. (These are the capillaries that bleed when you cut your finger or "skin your knee.") The epidermal cells at the very botom layer receive a rich supply of food materials and oxygen. But the cells in the layers farther out do not have any direct contact with the blood capillaries. They are starved more and more, the closer to the surface they go. Gradually they die, and their cell proteins are changed into a horny substance called *keratin* (KER-UH-TIN). The flattened, dead epidermal cells form a tough *keratin layer* that covers all the outer body surfaces. This layer is a key part of the wall around us. It helps to keep invading bacteria out, and also helps keep fluids from evaporating out of the more delicate living tissues below. Without the dead keratin layer of the skin, the living epidermis would quickly dry out and crack.

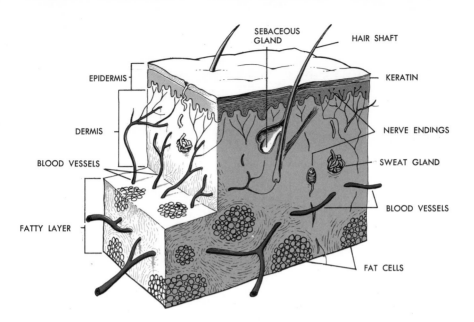

A section of the skin.

The epidermis is made up of a number of layers of cells, but each is so tiny that the epidermis itself is quite thin. On most of your body the epidermis may be only a hundredth of an inch thick. On your eyelids it is even thinner. But in some other parts of the body, where special protection is needed, the keratin layer of the skin is much thicker. The soles of the feet are covered by a rather thick layer of keratin, and it grows even thicker if you go barefoot.

In places where there is an unusual amount of pressure on the skin, a tough, horny patch called a *callus* will build up. Calluses may form when shoes that do not fit properly press on the feet.

Corns may form on toes for the same reason. Many remedies are sold for removing calluses and corns, but they cannot solve the problem alone. If the shoe is still pressing on the foot in the same place, the callus or corn will form all over again. It is the skin's way of protecting itself from injury.

Pick up a pencil and hold it as though you were going to write. Now look at your middle finger, in the place where the pencil rested against it. Is there a small, thickened lump? You may find that this little lump grows larger during the school year, when you have to write down many notes and reports, but then it may disappear during the summer, when you do not use a pencil or pen very much. Your epidermis is adjusting its thickness according to the strain you are putting on it.

Have you ever met anyone who claimed to be able to read your fortune in your palm? When you look at the palm of your hand, you see many lines and creases. Some go across the palm, some slant up or down, and some form a network of criss-crossing lines. If you fold your hand inward, you will see that the large creases permit the extra skin of your palm to fold up neatly. The smaller lines (some are so small that you may need a magnifying glass to see them clearly) provide friction ridges, raised ribs of epidermis that make it easier to hold onto things than it would be if the palms of the hands were completely smooth and slippery.

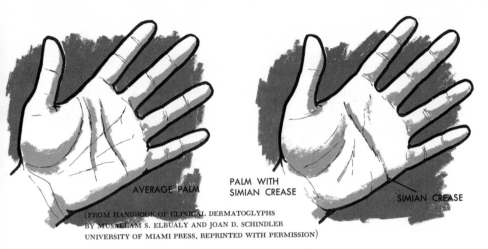

A "lifeline" in your palm.

Do the lines in your palm really tell anything about what your life will be like? Most people do not believe this. But recently it has been discovered that unusual palm prints may be linked with diseases and deformities. For example, look at the lines that run across your palm. Do you have a single large crease running from one side of your palm to the other? Or are there two large creases parallel to each other, neither of which runs completely across your hand? Only fourteen percent of people have a single large crease. (It is called a *simian crease,* because monkeys and apes generally have this kind of palm pattern.) But among babies that are born malformed, because their mothers caught German measles while they were pregnant, about fifty percent have a simian crease.

If you look at your fingertips, you will find patterns of friction ridges even more complicated than those on your palms. You can examine them more easily if you press each of your fingertips in turn on an ink pad, and then onto a clean sheet of paper. Are all your fingerprints the same? You may have heard that no two people in the world have exactly the same set of fingerprints. This is quite true, as far as scientists know, although some identical twins have fingerprints that are nearly alike.

Though your ten fingerprints are not exactly the same as anybody else's, you will find that each of them falls into one of four main types. These are the arch, the loop, the whorl, and the composite (a mixture of loops and forks). Your fingerprints have had the same pattern since five or six months be-

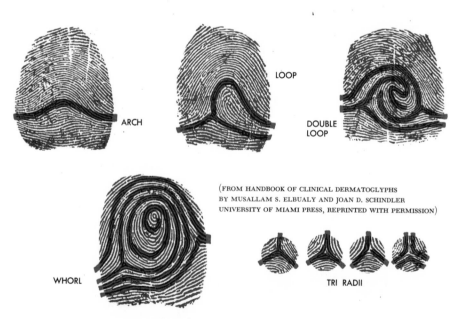

LOOP

ARCH

DOUBLE
LOOP

WHORL

(FROM HANDBOOK OF CLINICAL DERMATOGLYPHS
BY MUSALLAM S. ELBUALY AND JOAN D. SCHINDLER
UNIVERSITY OF MIAMI PRESS, REPRINTED WITH PERMISSION)

TRI RADII

Main classes of fingerprint patterns.

fore you were born, and—except for scars that might result from an accident—they will stay the same all your life.

Because each person has a unique set of fingerprints, which belong to nobody else on earth, they are a useful form of identification. A visible fingerprint might be left at the scene of a crime in the form of a smudge of blood or ink. But this does not happen very often. Police are more likely to find latent prints. These fingerprints are impressions left by the natural oils of the skin on some object. They cannot be seen with the naked eye, but when the detective dusts a bit of powder on them, they suddenly appear. A fine white powder, like talcum powder, is used to bring out fingerprints on a dark surface, such as a tabletop. Powdered graphite (the black "lead" in a lead pencil) is used for light surfaces. Smooth and shiny surfaces—a glass or doorknob, for example—give the best fingerprints. Rough surfaces or very porous one (like a paper towel) may not show any fingerprints at all. After photographing the fingerprints, the police detectives can compare them with the prints of likely suspects.

Try pressing your finger on a clean mirror. You may be able to make out a faint smudge, but you probably will not be able to see many details. Sprinkle a bit of talcum powder on the mirror.

With a feather or a soft tissue, very gently brush off the excess powder. Now you will see your fingerprint clearly outlined. The bits of powder stick to the oily smudges left by the ridges of your epidermis.

The epidermis is not the whole skin. Beneath it there is another, thicker layer, called the *dermis*. It is twenty to thirty times thicker than the epidermis. The epidermis and the dermis do not lie one on top of the other like two flat sheets of paper. Instead, the boundary between them is wavy. Bumps in the epidermis fit into hollows in the dermis, and vice versa.

The dermis contains various structures, including blood vessels, nerves, and special sense organs. If you pinch your skin or touch a hot pot, you feel it because of the sense organs and nerves in your dermis.

Have you ever had a hive or a skin rash? It may have been an *allergic* (AL-LUR-JIK) reaction. Special chemicals in your skin, called *antibodies*, reacted with chemicals called *antigens*, introduced from outside the body. After they combined, a chemical called *histamine* (HISS-TA-MEEN) was released. Histamine causes fluid to leak out of the blood vessels in the skin, making the tissues swell. The blood vessels widen, too, and they make the skin look red. Skin rashes can be caused by antigens in the things that come in contact with the skin, such as wool, poison ivy, or dishwashing detergents. Skin rashes can also be caused by an allergy to a food that is eaten or to a drug such as penicillin. Allergies can be treated with drugs called *antihistamines*, which block the effect of histamine. A series of injections of small amounts of the antigen can desensitize the body, or stop it from reacting to the antigen so strongly. Most people with allergies to a particular food or fabric simply try to avoid any contact with it.

Look how smoothly your skin covers all parts of your body. Pinch up a "tent" of skin from the inner part of your forearm. Now let it go. The skin of your arm is soft and smooth again. It fits snugly over your arm, with no sign that it had been stretched out. Elastic fibers in the dermis permit your skin to stretch to cover you, no matter how you may move the parts of your body. The network of elastic fibers in the dermis gives skin its toughness and strength.

Sweat glands are important structures in the dermis. They are found all over the body, but are particularly numerous in the armpits and the palms of the hands. These glands pour out moisture and help keep us cool.

Another kind of gland in the dermis is the *oil* or *sebaceous* (SEH-BAY-shus) *glands*. As you can

15

guess, these glands secrete oil, which helps to keep the skin smooth and soft. The sebaceous glands are usually wrapped around the base of *hair follicles* (FOLL-ih-kulz), which hold the "roots" of the hairs.

The living, growing parts of the hairs are found in the dermis. The thin hair shafts that grow out through the epidermis are mostly made of keratin. It does not hurt when you cut your hair, because the cells that form the hair shafts are dead. But it does hurt to pull a hair out by the root, for then you are tearing the living part, down in the dermis.

Deposits of fat are also found in the dermis, and in the layer of *subcutaneous* (sub-cue-TAYN-ee-us) *tissue* at the bottom of the dermis. These fatty deposits can act as cushions to protect us from pressure and bumps. (The two fatty cushions in the place where you sit down can help to protect you from spankings.) In cold weather, they act as blankets of insulation that help to keep us warm. They can also act as emergency food reserves for the body. Occasionally you may read in the newspaper about someone who was lost on an icy mountainside and had survived amazingly for many days without food until being rescued. Most often, these lucky survivors are either women (who have more subcutaneous fat deposits than men) or were a bit overweight before the emergency.

What color is your skin? If you are "white," you have undoubtedly noticed that your skin is not really white at all, but more like a sort of orangey, pinky, cream color. (You find out just how difficult it is to describe skin color when you try to mix paints to copy it.) If you are "black," your skin probably is not black at all—it may be a light tan color, or a brown color like coffee or chocolate. In fact, your skin may actually be lighter than the skin of some "white" people. Perhaps you are a "redskin"—but you know that your skin is not really red. And the skin of people of oriental ancestry is certainly not as yellow as a buttercup.

The color of skin is produced by colored chemicals called *pigments,* and we all—white, black, brown, red, or yellow—have the same basic set of pigments. There is the brown *melanin* (MELL-A-NIN), which is scattered through the epidermis. There is a yellow-orange pigment called *carotene* (KAR-OH-TEEN), which is found in the fatty parts of the skin. The blood pigments of *hemoglobin* inside the skin blood vessels also help to give skin its color.

The most important of the skin pigments is melanin. Blacks, as you might expect, have more melanin in their skin than whites do. This pigment is produced in special cells called *melanocytes* (MELL-A-NOH-SYTES) and then granules of melanin pass into other cells of the epidermis. Albinos are born without one of the key chemicals used in the melanocytes to make melanin. They cannot produce any of this pigment at all. Their skin is a pale pinkish color, and since hair and eye color is produced mainly by melanin also, albinos have nearly colorless hair and pink eyes. (The pink color comes from the pigments in the blood vessels behind the iris of the eye.)

When your skin is exposed to the sun, the melanin granules in your epidermis darken, and new melanin is produced in addition. Too much sun when you are not used to it may produce a painful sunburn. But if you build up your exposure to the sun gradually, you can develop a good suntan. How dark you will get depends on how much melanin you skin is capable of producing, and this is usually determined by heredity.

In some people the melanin is not scattered evenly through the epidermis. Instead, it occurs in little patches that produce dark-colored *freckles*. In the sun, the skin of these people does not tan very much. Instead, they get more freckles, while the skin around the freckles may still be quite light.

The sun can also produce dark spots on the skin called "liver spots." Other dark melanin-containing spots on skin are called *moles*. Moles are usually slightly raised, and they may have hairs growing

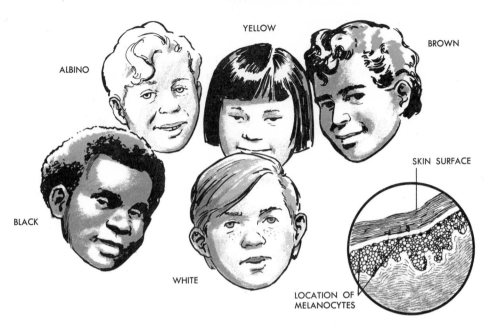

ALBINO

YELLOW

BROWN

BLACK

WHITE

SKIN SURFACE

LOCATION OF MELANOCYTES

Melanocytes in the skin determine skin color.

from them. Babies do not have any moles, but they gradually appear as a person grows. The average young adult has between forty and eighty moles. Moles can be removed by a doctor, but usually it is best to let them alone, unless they are very unsightly. Occasionally a mole can turn into a cancer —a mole that suddenly changes color or begins to bleed should be seen by a doctor quickly.

Warts are horny, raised patches of skin that do not contain melanin. They are caused by a virus, and like other conditions caused by germs, they can be spread from one person to another. They are most commonly found on the hands, and sometimes on the face. A person may have dozens of

19

them. There are many superstitions associated with warts—for example, that you can catch them by touching a frog or toad (because its skin is "warty"). Some "magic formulas" for getting rid of warts actually seem to work. But that is because warts often disappear by themselves, without any treatment. A doctor can offer much more reliable cures for warts than any "magic" rituals.

The melanin in your skin helps to screen out the ultraviolet rays of the sun, which might otherwise harm your body. Albinos must be very careful to avoid much exposure to sunlight, for they have no melanin to protect them.

Horny keratin, oil glands, sweat glands, blood vessels, nerves and sense organs, hairs, fat, pigments—the skin is much more than just a simple "rubber suit" that covers the body. Let's find out more about what it does for us and how it does its jobs.

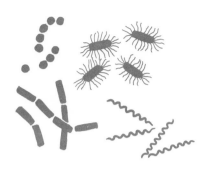

3

Skin for Defense and Stability

Your body is constantly in a state of siege. Outside an invading army waits, ready to take advantage of the slightest gap in your defenses, to sweep in and spread destruction it its wake.

The army is an invisible army, made of microbes too small to see without a micoscope. Millions of them swarm on your skin. Bathing does not remove them all, and each object you touch, even the air, brings new hordes of bacteria and viruses to you.

Your skin is your first line of defense against microbe invaders, and it is usually an effective one. The skin's defensive weapons begin before the skin itself is reached. The outer layer of the epidermis is evenly covered with a thin surface film. Water and various chemicals from the sweat glands and oils and other substances from the sebaceous glands all contribute to the skin's protective film. This amazing mixture can neutralize acids and bases, interfere with the absorption of poisons through the skin, and kill germs.

After the surface film comes the physical barrier of the tough, horny keratin layer. Bacteria, fungi, and various parasites are kept out of the body by the keratin layer, as long as it is not cracked or torn. Most chemicals are unable to pass through. There are a few important exceptions. Mercury spilled on the skin can pass through it to poison the body. So can some potent insecticides. Methyl salicylate is another chemical that can penetrate through unbroken skin. This chemical is often used in liniments that are smeared on the skin over painful, strained muscles. The chemical solvent dimethyl sulfoxide (DMSO) can not only pass through unbroken skin, but can also carry other chemicals along with it. DMSO seemed to be an unusually safe substance, and doctors hoped that it might be used to administer a great variety of drugs. It was widely used in the treatment of bursitis (a painful muscle condition) and other ailments, until reports began to come in that DMSO might cause changes in the eyes. Research on the use of DMSO is still going on, though now under very strict controls.

Recently there have been heated debates about another chemical that can pass through unbroken skin. This is hexachlorophene, a germ-killer that was widely used in deodorant soaps, shampoos, and antiseptics. Hospitals regularly bathed newborn babies in a preparation containing 3% hexachlorophene, and doctors and nurses also used this preparation to wash their hands. Then studies showed that baby monkeys bathed with the hexachlorophene preparation developed brain damage. The chemical was also found in blood samples from human babies who were bathed with the preparation. Quickly the Food and Drug Administration advised hospitals to stop using hexachlorophene preparations to bathe babies. But then a number of hospitals reported outbreaks of dangerous *Staphylococcus* infections after they stopped using the germ-killer.

A cut or scrape or burn can break into the skin's defenses. Immediately the bacteria that normally live on the skin, and others that might chance to be there, invade the body. The damaged tissues give off chemical messengers that summon white blood cells to the spot. A fierce battle takes place. The white cells swarm over the bacteria and eat them, only to die in turn, killed by poisons from the microbes. The dead bodies of the white cells pile up to form pus, which is a sign of infection. Careful cleaning of a wound and the application of germicides can cut down the danger of infection. Many doctors believe, though, that some common germicides, such as iodine, should not be used when the skin is broken, for they may damage the delicate living layers of the skin along with the germs.

Given a fair chance, the skin's ability to repair itself is amazing. Quickly, blood clots seal off the torn blood vessels. Cells in the neighboring tissues are stimulated to multiply, and soon they begin to invade the gap. Under the protective scab, new layers of skin cells are formed, elastic fibers knit together, and within days the scab falls off and there is a fresh pink coat of skin underneath. If the wound was very severe or the protecting scab was not allowed to remain long enough, the new skin

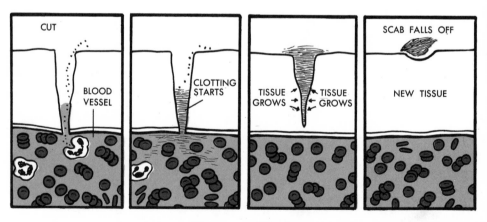

How a cut heals.

may be a tough connective-tissue *scar,* which lacks the normal pigments and may not be as soft and supple as normal skin. But often the skin repairs itself so well that it is soon impossible to tell where the wound occurred.

Defense is one important job of the skin. Another is to help keep the body temperature even. Have you ever taken your temperature when you were not sick? It was probably very close to 98.6°F. Your body can keep this same temperature whether it is hot or cold outside. This ability to keep an even temperature is shared by all the mammals, from mice to elephants to men, and by birds, too. These animals are called *warm-blooded animals,* because they can keep their bodies warm even when it is cold outside. A snake or lizard cannot do this. Neither can a grasshopper or a clam, or any other animal that is not a mammal or a bird.

Warm-blooded animals have a great advantage in the struggle for life. Most of the enzymes of the body—special proteins that help other body chemicals to react—work best at a temperature of just about 99°F. If the temperature is much lower, the chemical reactions of the body slow down. A *cold-blooded animal,* which cannot control its own body temperature, becomes sluggish in cold weather. If the temperature drops too far, it must either

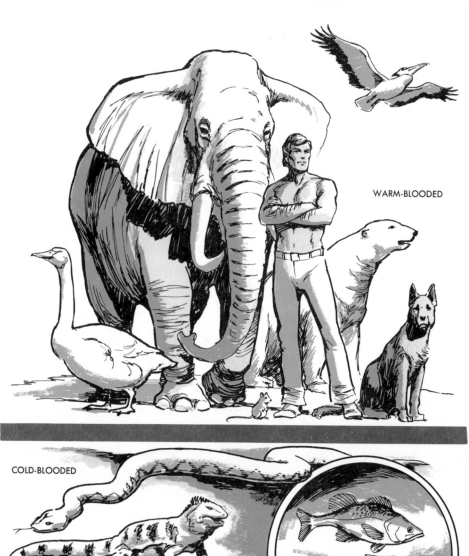

WARM-BLOODED

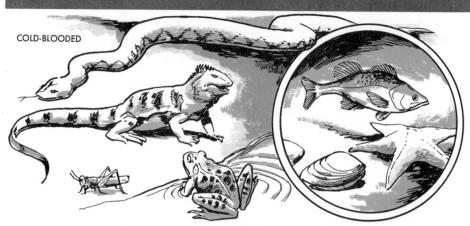

COLD-BLOODED

hibernate or die. But too high a temperature is not good for an animal, either. Enzymes are delicate chemicals; too much heat can damage or destroy them. A warm-blooded animal can keep its body temperature just right.

Temperature control in the body of a warm-blooded animal is a very delicate balance that results from a cooperation between the skin and special temperature-control centers in the brain. Sense organs in the skin, which are sensitive to heat and cold, send a constant stream of messages to the brain, keeping it informed of the temperature outside. When a change must be made, you do not have to think about it consciously. Your temperature-control centers take care of it automatically.

There are several different ways that the skin can raise or lower the temperature of the body. One important means of heat control is found in the blood vessels that carry blood through the skin. Blood is a watery liquid, and water has some unusual abilities. Have you ever waited for a pot of water to boil? You probably noticed that it took a long time. At first the water just got hotter and hotter, but it still stayed liquid. Scientists have found that water can hold a great deal of heat, much more than most other substances.

Many of the chemical reactions in the body cells

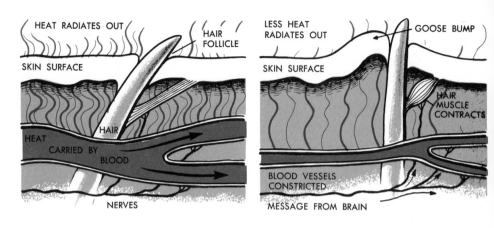

The skin helps to cool and warm the body.

produce heat. Muscle cells, in particular, produce a great deal of heat when they contract. And some muscle cells are contracting all the time, even when you are not walking or moving about. If all this heat were allowed to build up in the cells, they soon would become so hot that their enzymes and other important chemicals would be damaged. Eventually they would die. Instead, the heat produced by the body cells is picked up by the water in the blood moving through the blood vessels. In its travels through the body, this blood passes through blood vessels close to the surface of the skin. Heat tends to move from warmer things to cooler things. Since the outside air is usually cooler than the body, heat radiates out through the blood vessel walls, through the layers of skin cells, and out into the air.

But what if it is *very* cold outside? Heat may radiate out faster than it is produced by the body cells. If this were allowed to continue, the whole body would quickly cool down. The temperature-control centers in the brain do not allow this to happen. As soon as the skin sense organs send messages indicating a dangerous loss of heat, the temperature-control centers in turn send messages along nerves back to the skin. These messages tell the blood vessels in the skin to narrow, or constrict. Not as much blood can flow through constricted blood vessels, and so there is less loss of heat.

Other messages from the brain center cause tiny muscles attached to the hair follicles to contract. Their action causes the body hairs to stand up. That is the cause of the "goosebumps" that you get in cold weather. Your body hair is so short and sparse that this is not a very effective heat-conserving measure for you. But it works very well for an animal, like a cat or dog that has a thick coat of fur. A layer of air, heated by radiation from the body, is trapped in the thick fur and acts like an insulating blanket that helps to keep the animal warm. When the hairs stand up, a thicker air blanket is trapped among them and thus provides better insulation.

Messages from the temperature-control centers also cause some of the muscles to contract very rapidly. This is shivering, and it helps to warm the body with the extra heat produced by muscle action.

Have you ever noticed that you feel much colder when a wind is blowing than when the air is still? If cool air moves past your skin, it carries away the layer of warm air next to your body, and more warmth is radiated out. The larger the skin surface you have, the more heat you lose. You can test this principle with a simple experiment. Heat up some water and pour eight ounces into a cup and another eight ounces of hot water onto a dinner plate. Allow both to stand, and measure the temperature of the water from time to time. (You can use a thermometer—not the kind you use to take your temperature, but a larger one, which goes up past the boiling point of water. Or you can simply feel the water with your finger.) You will find that the water on the dinner plate, with a much larger surface, cools down much faster than the water in the cup.

The amount of skin surface you have depends on the way your body is built. A tall thin person has more skin surface than a short fat person with the same weight. If you find this hard to believe, test it with two sets of six square blocks. Pile one set of blocks one on top of another, so that you have a single tower six blocks high. Stack the other set of blocks in two columns next to each other, three blocks high. Now count the number of block surfaces exposed to the air. In the single tower, if you count the surface resting on the ground, twenty-six surfaces are exposed to the air. In the shorter, fatter, double tower, only twenty-two surfaces are exposed, even though both sets of blocks have exactly the same weight. A tall, thin person therefore loses heat in cold weather faster than a short, fat person of the same weight, and he may need to wear heavier clothing to keep warm. (The short, fat person also has more fat deposits to help keep him warm, of course.)

What happens when it is very warm outside? Heat must still be carried away from the body cells, but now it cannot radiate out through the skin. For

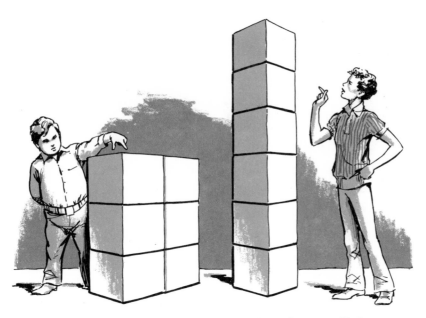

A short fat person has less skin surface than a tall thin person of the same weight.

the air is nearly as warm as or even warmer than the skin surface.

Now the body is aided by another unusual property of water. If you place a thermometer in a pan of water on a stove, you will find that the temperature rises steadily for awhile, until it reaches 212°F. Then the temperature of the water stays at the same value, as the water finally begins to boil. If you boil the water all the way down to the bottom of the pot, its temperaure will still stay at 212°F. Before the water boiled, the heat that the stove put into it was being used to change it from a liquid to a vapor. Water vapor can carry off an enormous amount of heat when it evaporates.

The sweat glands are the skin's means of evaporating water out into the air. Did you know that you are sweating all the time? Normally you can't see the sweat, because it is carried off immediately as an invisible gas. This kind of sweating can take care of the body's cooling needs very well when the air around you is dry. But if it is very humid, the air cannot hold more water vapor. Then the sweat runs along the body surface as a liquid. It carries away some heat, but not as much as it would if it could evaporate. In fact, too much sweating in hot, humid weather can even be harmful. Normally, you sweat out about a pint of water a day. But if a person is doing hard work in a hot, humid place, he may lose as much as three quarts of water in twenty-four hours. The body cannot safely spare that much water. Nor can it do without the salts that the sweat carries away. That is why it is important to drink a large amount of water in hot weather, and to eat more salt than usual to replace what is lost by sweating.

When the skin temperature sense organs send messages indicating too much heat to the brain's temperature-control centers, messages quickly come back to the skin to produce a widening or dilation of the skin blood vessels and an increase in sweating. The skin may become too hot when the air outside the body is hot, and also during hard work or heavy exercise. (During exercise, extra heat is produced by the contractions of the muscle cells.) Try running quickly up a flight of stairs, and then feel various parts of your skin for moisture. Although sweat glands are spread over nearly all parts of your body, you will probably find that you are sweating most in certain areas—perhaps your underarms, your scalp, forehead, neck, and back.

Heat is not the only thing that can make a person sweat. When a big-league baseball player goes up to bat, he generally scoops up a handful of dirt to rub on the palms of his hands before he steps into the batter's box. The pitcher, too, may dry his hands before he goes into his windup and he may wipe his sleeve across his forehead. They are both nervous, and nervousness can suddenly make the sweat glands pour out moisture even if it is not hot. The sweat glands in the palms of the hands and the soles of the feet are particularly sensitive to nervousness and other emotions. The sweat glands in the underarms, the scalp and other parts of the body can also respond to emotions.

Indeed, emotions may have a great effect on the skin. Anger or embarrassment may cause the blood vessels in the skin to dilate suddenly, producing a crimson blush as the blood pigments shine through the skin. Great fear may cause your skin blood vessels to constrict, making your skin turn pale. Emotions may even cause the skin to break out into a rash that looks just like a rash caused by poison ivy or some irritating chemical. The concert pianist, William Kapell, broke out in a terrible rash before every concert. When it was actually time for him to play, he was able to conquer his nervousness and do his work well. After the concert was over, the mysterious rash would promptly disappear.

There are two types of sweat glands in the skin. One kind, the *eccrine* (EK-KRIN) *glands*, are found nearly everywhere on the body surface. The other type, the *apocrine* (AP-O-KRIN) *glands* are found mainly in the armpits, in the genital regions, and in

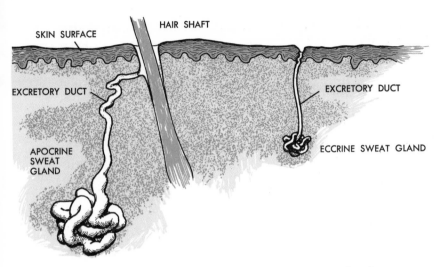

SKIN SURFACE

HAIR SHAFT

EXCRETORY DUCT

EXCRETORY DUCT

APOCRINE
SWEAT
GLAND

ECCRINE SWEAT GLAND

The body has two kinds of sweat glands.

the nose. The two types of sweat glands look rather similar. Each consists of a tightly coiled tube buried deep in the dermis, ending in a straighter portion through which the sweat flows out. The apocrine sweat glands are usually larger than the eccrine glands, and they generally empty into a hair follicle. The smaller eccrine glands send their sweat out directly to the outside, through openings in the epidermis called *pores*.

Eccrine sweat is a clear, watery substance that is ninety-nine percent water. The other one percent is made up of dissolved salt and waste materials. The waste materials in sweat are very similar to those found in urine, but urine is much more concentrated.

Apocrine sweat is a milky white, sticky substance. This is the kind of sweat that all the underarm deodorant commercials are aimed at. It contains a number of smelly substances, and its odor is made even stronger by the fact that bacteria find apocrine sweat very nourishing and multiply in it. Frequent washing of the armpits and other areas where apocrine glands are concentrated can help to cut down unpleasant "body odors."

Actually, before puberty, children do not have to worry much about body odors, for their apocrine glands are not very active. Their sweat does not contain the same chemicals as the sweat of adults, and the assortment of bacteria that live on children's skin is usually quite different from the skin bacteria of adults. As a result, children smell different from adults.

Indeed, each person has his own personal "smell signature," which is not exactly the same as anyone else's. If you have a pet dog, he recognizes you even when he can't see you by your own characteristic smell. Your "smell signature" is made up of a combination of the air you breathe out, and the secretions of your oil and sweat glands. Sometimes, when a person is ill, special chemicals give a particular odor to his personal smell. It is said that an experienced doctor can diagnose many diseases with clues from the way his patients smell. Scientists are now trying to analyze the chemicals that make up a "smell signature" with very sensitive chemical gas analyzers. They are comparing the smell patterns of healthy people and people with various diseases. They hope that some day an automatic machine will be able to diagnose illnesses by analyzing the smell patterns that the patient gives off.

Some glands of the body are really special types of apocrine sweat glands. The *cerumen* (SEH-ROO-MEN) *gland*, which produces ear wax, is a type of apocrine gland. The *mammary glands* are specialized apocrine glands that produce nourishing milk instead of sweat. These glands develop fully only in women, and normally they do not actually secrete milk until a woman has had a baby.

The sebaceous glands in the skin grow out of the epithelium of the hair follicle. They look like small clusters of grapes, and they empty their secretions into the channel in which the hair root grows.

The substance that sebaceous glands secrete is called *sebum* (SEE-BUM). It is a waxy substance that is spread over the surface of the skin by sweat. Sebum helps to keep the skin from drying out, and it helps to keep the hair from becoming dry and brittle.

Take a handful of your hair and rub it between your fingers. Now rub your fingers over your scalp.

Which seemed oilier? Now run a brush through your hair one hundred times. Brushing helps to spread sebum over the hair. Does your hair feel any oilier after brushing? Does it look shinier? When a bird preens itself, it is doing something very similar. It is spreading oil from its sebaceous glands over its feathers.

Scientists have found much evidence to indicate that the secretions of the sebaceous glands are controlled both by nerves and by endocrine glands. During puberty, when the sex organs are developing and a child is changing into a man or woman, there are many changes in the glands of the body. Sometimes the seabaceous glands may begin to work overtime, producing more oil than is needed. As a result, the skin and hair may become oily and harder to keep clean. Some bacteria find the waxy sebum nourishing, and they may grow and multiply on oily skin. These bacteria result in unsightly blackheads, pimples, and other small skin infections. This condition is called *acne* (AK-NEE), and it is very common among teenagers. Most people have only a few troublesome pimples or blackheads, but some teenagers may have stubborn infections of the sebaceous glands that may even leave permanent scars on the face and upper back. Frequent washing to remove the buildup of oil and bacteria is very important in controlling acne. A poor diet, lack of sleep, and tension (for example,

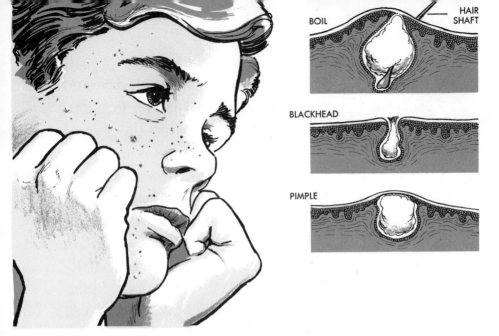

Oil and bacteria can build up in pores and cause skin problems.

worrying about exams) can cause an acne attack to flare up. Squeezing pimples with your fingers can spread the infection and make things worse. The more severe cases of acne should be treated by a doctor.

One thing that doctors do not all agree about is how much sun is good for people. Certainly everyone agrees that a bad sunburn never did anybody any good. But what about sunbathing? Many people believe that people who are out in the sun a lot are healthier than people who stay indoors most of the time. Up to a certain point, this may be true.

But too much sun can be very bad for the skin. Sunrays can damage the elastic fibers in the dermis and make the skin wrinkled and old looking. Too much exposure to sun can make skin dry and leathery. (These effects occur mainly in light-skinned people. The extra melanin in the skin of dark-skinned people screens out sunrays and helps to protect their skin.) Having skin that looks old when you are still relatively young is bad enough, but too much sun can have even more dangerous effects: it can cause skin cancer. Scientists can produce skin cancer in mice by exposing a particular area of their skin to light rays. Of course, experiments like this could not be tried on humans, but it has been found that people who work outdoors, such as farmers and sailors, have skin cancer more often than people who stay indoors most of the time. And at seaside resorts and other places where there is a great deal of sunlight and few clouds, the skin cancer rate is also higher than in regions where people are not exposed to the sun as much.

One benefit of sunbathing has been established definitely. Skin contains a fatty substance that is changed into a form of vitamin D when it is exposed to sunlight. This is an important vitamin for building strong bones and teeth. During the summer, when people are outdoors a great deal and wear little clothing, their skin makes plenty of vitamin D. Cows' milk produced in the summer is also rich in vitamin D, for cows' skin can make this vitamin, too. But in the wintertime, people stay indoors much of the time and wear heavy clothing that covers most of their bodies when they do go out. Cows, too, stay in the barn where it is warm. As the winter goes on, the body uses up its store of the "sunshine vitamin." Before this was discovered, children often got a disease called rickets. Their bones became soft and bent out of shape. After it was found that vitamin D could cure and prevent rickets, it became the custom to give children a daily dose of fish liver oil. (This oil is a rich source of the vitamin.) Now vitamin D is regularly added to milk and some other foods, so that everyone is sure to have enough of the "sunshine vitamin," all year round.

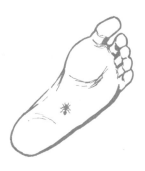

4
The Skin Senses

Close your eyes. Have someone place an object in front of you, without telling you what it is. Now touch the object with your fingertips. Feel its shape and texture. Try to guess what it is without opening your eyes. You will be surprised at how much you can find out about the world without using your eyes.

Special sense organs are found in the skin all over your body. Some of these sense *receptors* are sensitive to the slightest contact with the skin. These are the touch receptors. If an ant crawls over your leg, you will feel it, even though it weighs far less than a postage stamp. Several different kinds of sense receptors in the skin are sensitive to touch.

Some of the touch receptors are the bare ends of nerves, which branch out through the epidermis.

If the ant stepped on a part of your epidermis containing one of these bare nerve endings, a message would immediately travel down the nerve and then along a chain of other nerves to the brain. As soon as your brain interpreted the message, you would have a feeling that there was something on your leg. If you decided to do something about it, your brain would send messages to the muscles of your hand and arm, directing them to move your hand down to brush the ant off.

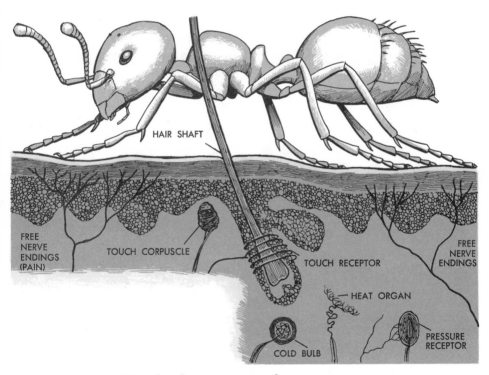

The skin has a variety of sense organs.

The ant might set off another type of "touch alarm" by bumping into one of the small hairs on your leg. A nerve ending is wrapped around the bottom of each hair follicle. If anything touches the hair and moves it slightly, a message is sent to inform the brain. This type of touch receptor can work even before an object actually touches the skin. It is a sort of "early warning system" that might be useful in informing you of a mosquito coming in for a landing before it has had a chance to bite you. Animals use this kind of touch receptor more than humans do. The whiskers of a cat or mouse are stiff hairs with nerve endings wrapped around their follicles. A mouse carefully checks the size of a hole with its whiskers before crawling through it.

Some sense receptors in the skin do not respond at all to a light touch, but they do respond to a stronger pressure. Other receptors are stimulated both by touch and by pressure, but they send different messages to the brain, so that you know just how strong the touch was.

A third type of skin sense is provided by the pain receptors. You probably think of pain as a bad thing, but actually it is a very important means of protection for the body. Pain is a warning that something is wrong—that damage is being done to the body, or may be done, unless immediate action is taken. Often the brain or spinal cord takes care of the action automatically, before you have even been informed of the situation. If you touch a hot pot, for example, your pain receptors are stimulated, and immediately messages are sent to the brain by way of the spinal cord. If you had to wait until the brain interpreted all the messages, figured out where the pain was coming from, decided what to do, and then sent messages to the right muscles, you would wind up with a bad burn. Fortunately, the spinal cord can send its own messages immediately to make you move your hand away from the pot. This type of quick reaction is called a *reflex action*. By the time the messages are interpreted in your brain and you realize the danger, a reflex action has already removed your hand from the pot.

Many things can stimulate pain receptors. Hard pressure, great heat or cold, certain chemicals, an electric shock—all can give us a sensation of pain. A cut or scrape, or anything else that damages tissues will make us feel pain, as long as these tissues have their share of pain receptors. (There are some places inside the body that have very few pain receptors, or none at all. Surprisingly, the brain itself is one of these places.)

The pain receptors are designed not to give us "false alarms." A light stimulation of a pain receptor will not produce any sensation at all. Only a pain stimulus of a certain strength will cause a feeling of pain. Scientists call this value the *pain threshold*. If a stimulus is just over the pain threshold, we feel a tickling sensation. A little stronger stimulus may cause an annoying itch. And a stronger stimulus still will produce a feeling of pain.

Some people react to pain much more strongly than others. The pain of a bad cut may make one person cry or even vomit, while another person with the same kind of cut may not show much sign of suffering. Scientists believe that our reaction to pain depends on how many messages are sent to various parts of the brain after the first pain signals are received. How you react to pain probably depends partly on the kind of brain and nervous system you were born with, and partly on how you were brought up to respond to things in general.

There are some other unusual things about the pain receptors. If your touch receptors are stimulated, your brain knows exactly where the messages came from. If there is a fly on your arm, you can brush it away without even bothering to look at it. But pain messages are more general. If the brain had only the messages from the pain receptors to go on, it might know, for example, only that a mosquito was biting you somewhere on the upper half of your left arm, but not exactly where. Fortunately, this is not usually too great a handicap. For most things that stimulate pain receptors on the skin also stimulate touch receptors at the same time.

Most of the sense organs have the ability to adapt to a stimulus that continues for a long time, and after awhile they stop sending messages to the brain. This is a lucky thing. If your touch receptors were unable to adapt to continuing stimuli, for example, you would never be able to wear clothes. You would constantly have the feeling that something was pressing on you. Even the touch of the hair on your head would drive you crazy. The heat and cold receptors in your skin also can adapt to stimuli. A hot tub soon feels comfortable even if the water has not cooled down very much. A swimming pool that feels icy when you first plunge in quickly stops stimulating your cold receptors. But pain receptors are different. As long as the painful stimulus keeps up, your pain receptors will continue sending messages to your brain at the same strength. Can you think of an advantage in having them work that way?

The heat and cold receptors of your skin work together with pain receptors to provide you with a built-in thermometer. You can tell just by feeling something whether it is hotter than your body

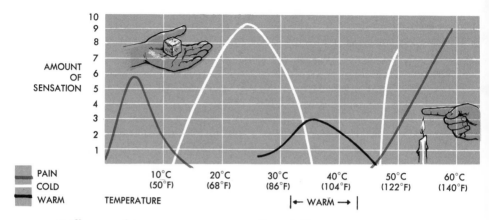

Different skin receptors respond in different temperature ranges.

temperature, or colder. If you touch something cool, your cold receptors are stimulated. But if you touch something that is very hot or cold, some peculiar things happen.

Did you ever pick up an ice cube and think that it felt burning hot? That was because of the odd way your skin temperature receptors and brain work together. Below a certain temperature (about 45°F), your cold receptors are not stimulated any more, but your pain receptors are. When the temperature goes down close to freezing, even the pain receptors do not respond any more—your skin becomes numb. When the temperature is very high, you would expect your heat receptors to respond more than ever. But this does not happen at all.

After about 115°F, your heat receptors do not respond any more. Instead, your pain receptors and your *cold* receptors are stimulated! No wonder your brain gets a little confused sometimes.

Your built-in thermometer usually works rather well. If you do not know whether or not to wear a jacket to school, you can stick your arm out the door and "feel" how cool it is. You can test a drop of your baby brother's milk on the thermal receptors of your wrist to see if it is just the right temperature. You can touch your lips to someone's forehead to see if he has a fever. Your temperature senses even work for you when you are sleeping. The skin of your body senses whether it is too warm or too cool in the room and without even waking up, you can kick off the covers or pull up an extra blanket.

The various skin sense receptors are spread over all parts of the body, but they are not spread evenly. The most sensitive parts of your skin are your fingertips and lips. On the tip of each one of your fingers, for example, there are about a hundred separate touch receptors. In other parts of the body there are far fewer. In the skin of your back, the touch receptors may be as much as two inches apart. You can test this for yourself. Have someone poke you in the back with one, two, or three fingers and try to guess how many fingers he used.

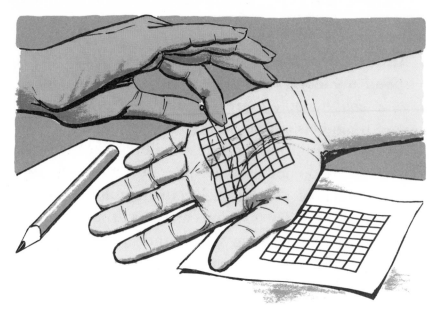

Mapping the skin senses.

You will probably think it was only one, unless he spread his fingers wide. Yet if he does the same thing on the back of your hand (with your eyes closed, so that you can't see how many fingers he is using), you probably will be able to tell easily.

You can make a map of your skin sense receptors. Mark off a checkerboard of tiny squares in black ink on the skin of some part of your body—the palm of your hand, your leg, or your back. Draw another checkerboard of the same size on a sheet of paper. Now have someone blindfold you and test each square for sense receptors. He can test for touch receptors by a very light touch with a wisp of cotton. For pressure receptors he can press firmly with the rounded head of a pin. If he presses gently with the point of the pin (not hard enough to break the skin), your pain receptors will be stimulated. He can test for heat and cold receptors by placing one metal fork in a bowl of hot water and another in a bowl of ice water, then touching one tine of the heated or cooled fork to each square on your skin. Each time you report a sensation, he should mark it down on the proper square of the paper checkerboard, using a different-colored dot for each skin sense. When he finishes, you will have a map that shows how the various sense receptors are spread through that particular patch of skin.

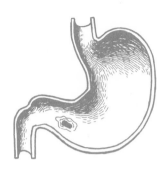

5

Linings

Do you know anyone who has an ulcer? He has a hole in the lining of his stomach. The acid juices in his stomach have actually burned away some of the epithelial cells that normally cover the inside of his stomach wall.

It seems amazing that this does not happen more often. Yet most people never get an ulcer. For the stomach actually has a double lining. There is a sheet of epithelial cells, and these in turn are covered by a slimy coat of mucus. The thick mucus coat protects the delicate cells of the stomach lining from the acid in the digestive juices.

The epithelial tissue of the stomach lining is composed of a number of different kinds of cells. Columnar cells form most of the covering sheet, but scattered among them are specialized cells that act as tiny glands. Some of them secrete the hydrochloric acid that helps to digest our food (and may cause an ulcer). Other cells produce other chemicals that aid in digestion. Vase-shaped goblet cells secrete the mucus that spreads over the stomach lining. If these cells do not produce enough mucus, the protective coat will be thin and the stomach acid will eat through the delicate epithelial tissue. The hole that is formed is an ulcer, and it can be extremely painful.

Doctors believe that if you are nervous and upset, you will increase your chances of getting an ulcer. Strong emotions can make the acid-secreting cells work overtime. They produce so much acid that even the mucus coating cannot provide enough protection. Strong emotions can also interfere with the work of the mucus-secreting cells, so that they do not produce enough of the protective coating. If an ulcer patient can be helped to calm down and does not eat foods that will irritate the sore spot even more, his stomach lining can gradually repair itself.

The lining of the stomach is part of a mucous membrane that stretches unbroken from the openings of the nose and mouth down the air and food passageways, lining all the tubes and air sacs of the lungs and the entire digestive tract down to the anus, the opening at the bottom of the trunk of the body. Each part of this membrane is covered

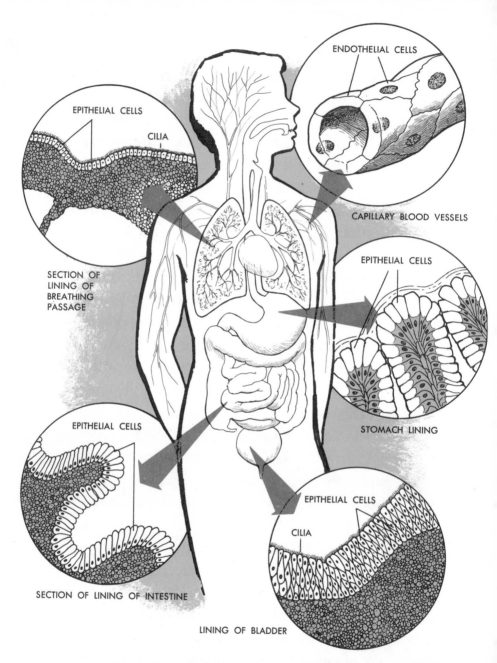

EPITHELIAL CELLS

ENDOTHELIAL CELLS

CILIA

CAPILLARY BLOOD VESSELS

SECTION OF
LINING OF
BREATHING
PASSAGE

EPITHELIAL CELLS

STOMACH LINING

EPITHELIAL CELLS

EPITHELIAL CELLS

CILIA

SECTION OF LINING OF INTESTINE

LINING OF BLADDER

Epithelial cells line the organs of the body.

with a slimy coat of mucus, which helps to protect the delicate tissues underneath. Special epithelial cells in each organ secrete chemicals or do other jobs that are needed.

In the small intestine, the mucus membrane lining is gathered into many circular folds, which increase the surface through which food materials can be absorbed. Fingerlike *villi* (VILL-EYE) project from the intestinal lining and increase the surface still more. Tiny gland cells secrete mucus or intestinal juices.

The lining of the breathing passages contains many ciliated epithelial cells. The tiny, hairlike cilia beat back and forth in rhythm and produce a current in the slimy mucus. The current always flows upward. The air that you breathe in may contain some solid dust particles. Many of these are screened out by the fringe of stiff hairs at the entrance to the nostrils. The solid particles that get past this first line of defense are caught in the sticky mucus further down, and are gradually pushed upward by the current. Eventually they reach a point where they can be coughed or sneezed out of the body.

The viruses and bacteria that cause colds can live and multiply in the passages of the nose, even though these passages are much cooler than the inner regions of the body, where many other kinds of bacteria thrive. When cold microbes are multiplying inside your nose, the mucous membranes become irritated. The lining may swell so much that it is difficult to get any air through your nose, and the mucus-secreting cells begin working overtime. They produce more mucus than is needed to coat the membrane, and the extra mucus drips out. The stuffy, runny nose that you have when you catch a cold results from your mucous membrane's fight against the microbes that have invaded it.

A separate mucous membrane lines the kidneys and bladder and the organs and passageways of the reproductive organs. Ciliated epithelial cells help to push the urine along. Ciliated cells in the sperm ducts of a man help to send his sperms out of the body. In a woman's Fallopian tubes, ciliated cells help to capture a ripe egg and send it down toward the uterus, where it may ultimately develop into a baby.

All the blood vessels of the body have their own epithelial lining. It is called *endothelium* (EN-DOH-THEEL-EE-UM). The endothelium is as thin a lining as you can get: only one cell thick. And it is as leaky as a sieve. Liquids and gases can pass through it easily. In fact, white blood cells can squeeze in and out through the walls of the capillaries. This is a very good thing, for it permits the white blood cells to patrol the tissues outside the blood vessels and capture and destroy invading bacteria wherever they might be.

Sometimes cholesterol and other fats are deposited in the linings of the blood vessels. These deposits may build up so much that they can nearly close a large artery. The deposits are rough, and they may tear the delicate blood platelets passing through them. The torn platelets spill out chemicals that cause blood clots to form. A blood clot may stick in a part of the artery that is already narrowed by fat deposits and plug it up completely. Then, depending on where the plugged artery is, a heart attack or a stroke may result.

Doctors believe that the Americans' diet is a main cause of the fat deposits that can lead to heart attacks. They think that we eat too much fat and sugar. They feel that we should have more protein in our diet, and cut down on fat and sugar. Meanwhile, they are experimenting on various drugs and surgical methods to remove fat deposits from the blood vessel linings and to prevent them from forming.

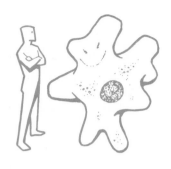

6
Coverings from Ameba to Man

Your skin helps to protect you, to keep you from drying out, and to keep you in touch with the world around you. All living creatures face the same kinds of problems and have needs very much like yours. All of them have outer coverings that do much the same jobs as your skin. But not all organisms have a covering that can really be called skin. Instead, scientists use a more general term, *integument* (IN-TEG-YEW-MENT), when they speak about the coverings of different kinds of organisms.

Your skin, for example, is made up of trillions of skin cells. An ameba or a paramecium cannot have a "skin" like that, for its entire body consists of just one cell. (It is a rather large cell, though—quite a bit larger than any of your skin cells.)

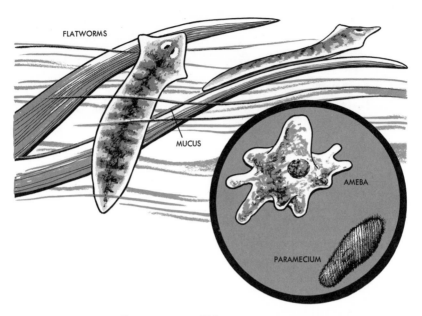

Tiny pond creatures all have an outer covering.

The ameba's integument is just a cell membrane, a covering very much like the membranes that surround each of your individual cells. The ameba's cell membrane holds its jellylike body together, but it is not stiff enough to keep a fixed shape. The ameba changes its shape constantly as it moves about and feeds on other small pond creatures. One part of its body will bulge out to form a "foot" to creep on, or a pair of "arms" to catch its prey. Water and chemicals can pass through the membrane, in and out of the ameba's one-cell body.

The paramecium's integument is a much more formal affair. It is stiffened to form a firm covering called a *pellicle* (PELL-ih-kul). It cannot change its shape as the ameba does, but keeps a slipperlike shape. The paramecium's pellicle is marked by an interesting pattern, which looks something like a honeycomb. A tiny hairlike cilium sticks up out of the bottom of each six-sided hollow in the pellicle. The paramecium uses its cilia to swim and to send a current of water into its mouth. It feeds on bacteria and other bits of matter carried in by the feeding current.

The flatworm has cilia on its integument, too. But the flatworm is a many-celled animal, and its covering is a real epithelium, made up of a single layer of cells. The flatworm's back is bare, but its belly surface is covered with cilia. It secretes a slimy mucus, and the cilia lash back and forth in this slimy liquid. The flatworm slides along like a gliding ribbon.

Starfish and sea urchins belong to a group called *echinoderms* (EE-KINE-oh-DERMZ), which means "spiny skin." Their integument is a hard, tough covering, reinforced by limy plates. Scattered over this outer covering are numerous spines, which give these animals their name.

You might think that a snail's shell is its "skin," but this is not so. The shells of snails and their two-shelled relatives, such as clams and oysters, are nonliving materials, which are formed by special "shell glands." The real integument of snails and their relatives is underneath their hard, limy shells, and it is an epidermis made of ciliated cells.

Insects have an outer covering called a *cuticle* (CUE-TIH-KUL) that is like a jointed suit of armor. It is made of a tough substance called *chitin* (KYE-TIN), which is secreted by the living epidermis underneath. The insect's cuticle fits it tightly and does not give it any room to grow. In order to grow, the insect must *molt*, or shed its cuticle.

When an insect is ready to molt, its epidermal cells secrete chemicals that are like digestive juices. These chemicals eat away the inside of the chitin coat and loosen it. The old cuticle splits, and the insect wriggles out. Its soft epidermis has been busy secreting a new chitin coat, along with all the

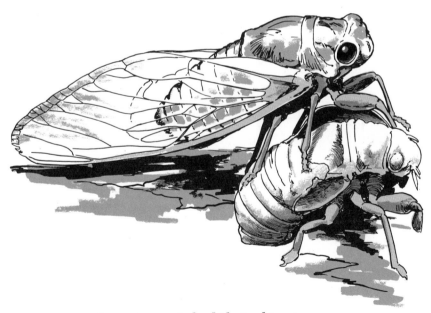

Insects must shed their skins to grow.

glands and sense organs that go with it. The epidermal cells can repair wounds and even regrow legs or other parts that the insect had lost before it molted. When the soft new cuticle is exposed to the air, it quickly hardens, and soon the insect is protected by a new, larger chitin coat.

The insect's protective covering does two jobs—it is both an integument and a skeleton-on-the-outside, which supports the insect's body and helps it to move. The group to which we humans belong is built according to a different plan. These are the *vertebrates,* animals with backbones. We all have a skeleton of bones on the inside of the body and a flexible skin on the outside that serves as an integument.

Although the skin of all the vertebrates follows the same basic plan, there are many differences depending on how the animal lives. A frog, for example, spends its whole life in or close to the water. It has a very thin skin, which must always be kept moist. The frog may actually "breathe" through its skin, exchanging oxygen and carbon dioxide with the gases dissolved in the thin film of moisture on its skin. From time to time, the frog will shed the outer layer of its epidermis, much as the insect sheds its cuticle.

Animals that live in desert regions, where water is scarce, have a much thicker skin, which cuts down the loss of water from the body. You may think of snakes as "slimy," but if you touch one, you will find that its skin is actually quite dry.

Many animals have deposits of melanin and other pigments in their skin. Some of them can change their color to match their surroundings or express an emotion. Usually this is done by expanding or contracting the pigmented cells, so that the entire skin looks darker or lighter. You may know that some lizards and fishes can change color to match their environment. But did you know that an octopus can blush? Its thin epidermis contains little flexible bags of blue, green, yellow, brown, or red pigments, which can change their shape to change the color of the octopus's skin. When it is excited, it may look like a constantly changing rainbow. If it is frightened, it may turn quite pale.

Colors in the integument serve many purposes in the animal world. Some animals use their colors as camouflage, blending almost perfectly with their surroundings. A green grasshopper is hard to see as it perches on green leaves. The wings of some moths are speckled with gray and brown and almost perfectly match the tree trunks on which the moths rest all day. The dappled spots on the back of a young fawn make him hard to see amid the patterns of sunlight and shadows of the thicket. When he is old enough to go out with his mother,

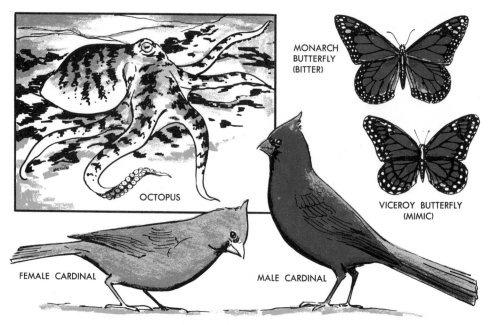

MONARCH
BUTTERFLY
(BITTER)

VICEROY BUTTERFLY
(MIMIC)

OCTOPUS

FEMALE CARDINAL

MALE CARDINAL

Animals use color in many ways.

he loses his baby spots and gets a coat of brown fur.

Some animals have such bright colors that they could never blend into their surroundings. It seems as though their colors are made to call attention to them. Many butterflies, for example, have brightly colored wings. Their colorful patterns are produced by many tiny colored scales. Some of these bright-colored butterflies are poisonous or bitter tasting. A bird that eats one by mistake quickly learns to avoid such butterflies in the future. In this case, color is used as a warning signal. It works so well that the color patterns of some bad-tasting butter-flies also appear on butterflies that are really good to eat. The birds cannot tell the difference and leave both kinds alone.

When a girl puts on a pretty dress to go out on a date, she is using color in a different way. Many animals, too, use pretty colors to attract a mate. Have you ever seen a peacock feather? The whole tail of the male peacock is full of these beautiful feathers, and he spreads them out as he struts in front of the female. Cardinals, bluebirds, and many other birds have brightly colored feathers that help them to win a mate. Usually the male is the brightly colored one. The female that he wins is generally dull in color, for she needs camouflage when she is sitting on her nest.

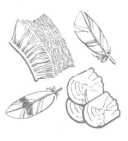

7

Feathers, Fur and Scales

Do you ever worry when you find hairs in your comb or brush? You may fear that you are going to get bald. But actually, there is nothing to worry about. Everyone loses hairs all the time—fifty to a hundred each day. These are hairs that have stopped growing and have been released by the hair follicles. After these follicles have rested awhile, they will begin to grow new hairs.

You have about a hundred thousand separate hairs on your head. Each one grows out of a hair follicle, set deep in the dermis. Hair begins as a living tissue. But, like the outer cells in your epidermis, the hair cells at the end of a growing hair soon die, and their proteins are changed into keratin. The hairs that you see growing out of your scalp are long tubes made of many keratinized hair cells, glued together.

Run your fingers lightly through your hair. Probably there will be a few hairs clinging to them when they come out. You did not feel any pain

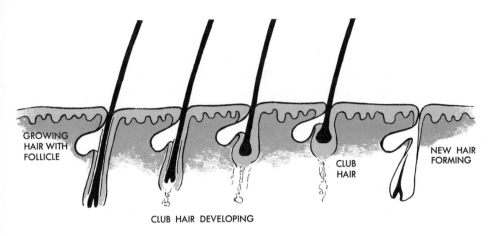

GROWING HAIR WITH FOLLICLE

CLUB HAIR DEVELOPING

CLUB HAIR

NEW HAIR FORMING

Life cycle of a hair.

when these hairs came out of your scalp, for they were already loose. Look closely at the ends of one of the hairs. You will see a small, whitish bulb, shaped like an onion bulb, at one end. This was the part that fiitted into the hair follicle. The bulb shape at the end shows that it had already stopped growing. Hair at this stage is called *club hair*.

Now take one of your firmly attached hairs and yank it out. That hurt! At the end of this hair, you will see a long whitish sheath, which came out of the hair follicle. This hair was still growing. It would not have come out if you had not pulled it.

Take a closer look at your hair. Is it straight or curly? Or perhaps it may be kinky (with very tight curls that spring back when you pull them and then let go), or woolly. What color is your hair? Are all your hairs the same color?

Look at the hair of your family and friends. Ask them for some samples, and compare them under a magnifying glass or microscope, if you can. You will discover that hairs are not all the same shape. Straight hairs look like straight tubes under a microscope. If you could cut a very thin cross section of a straight hair, you would find that it is perfectly round. Curly and kinky hairs are slightly flattened, with an oval cross section. There are pinches and bends along the length—this is what makes them spring into curls. Even if a curly-haired person has his hair straightened with chemicals in a beauty shop, these pinches and bends will still be in the hairs.

Under high magnification, you will discover that hairs are not the smooth, shiny tubes you thought they were. Each one is covered with tiny, overlapping scales. The scales are arranged in such a way that they lie flat if you brush your hair out from the scalp, but become ruffled if you brush the opposite way. Then your hair tangles more easily. That is how "teasing" hair by combing it the wrong way works. Take one of your hairs between your thumb and forefinger, and move them along the hair, first in one direction, then in the other. Which is easier?

What gives hair its color? Hair contains the pigment melanin, and the darker it is, the more melanin it contains. Red hair contains both melanin and a red pigment. You have probably guessed by looking at the people you know that hair color is inherited, just as skin color is. Light-haired parents usually have light-haired children. If one of the parents has very dark hair, there is a good chance that some or all of their children will be dark-haired too. If you know some cases that seem to break these rules, remember that some people change their hair color with dyes and bleaches.

Baldness runs in families, too. But you probably will not have to worry about going bald until you are middle-aged. And if you are a girl, you most likely will never go bald.

When you think of hair, you think first of the hair on you head. But nearly your whole body is covered with hair. There is hair on your arms and legs, on your chest and back, and on your face. Some of the hairs are so small you can hardly see them. Your eyelashes and eyebrows are special

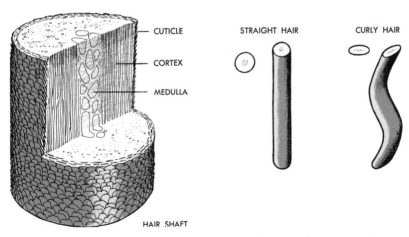

Microscopic views of human hair.

stiff hairs that help to protect your eyes. At puberty, boys and girls begin to grow coarse hairs in their underarms and genital regions. Men also have a coat of hair on their chests. If they do not shave each day, they will grow a beard and mustache on their faces.

Hair grows surprisingly quickly. The hairs on your head, for example, add about an inch in length each two-and-a-half months. (Hair growth usually speeds up a little in the summer and slows down in the winter.) But hairs do not go on growing indefinitely. Each type of hair seems to have built-in instructions that cause it to stop growing after a certain period. The hairs on your head grow for about two to six years, then they rest. Resting hairs tend to fall out easily, and so head hairs rarely grow more than three feet long. This is true whether you are a girl or a boy. Of course you can cut your hair long before it reaches that length. But you never cut your eyebrows or eyelashes. These hairs have such a short growing period that they never grow even an inch long. The hair on your body also stays quite short without being cut.

All our mammal relatives, from mice to elephants, have hair. Even a whale has some whiskers, and a baby whale has a full coat of fur before it is born. Most animals have a much longer and thicker coat of body hair than we humans do. The main function of an animal's fur is to trap a layer of air

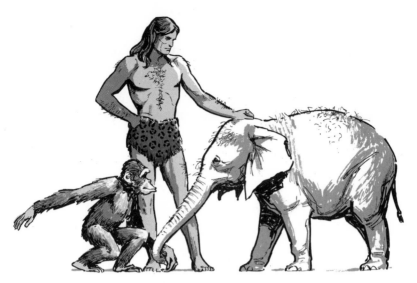

Mammals grow hair in various patterns.

next to the body, which keeps the animal warm But some mammals have special hairs that they use for other purposes. Did you know that a porcupine's quills are really a type of hair? The porcupine uses these stiff spines to defend itself from its enemies.

Birds do not have fur, but they have another type of "overcoat" that keeps them warm just as well. They have a coat of feathers.

A feather is an amazing structure. Hundreds of slender branches are attached to a long central shaft. Under a microscope you can see that these branches, called *barbs*, are like miniature feathers. Each one has many tiny branches, called *barbicels* (BAR-bih-sellz). Each barbicel is equipped with tiny hooks, which hold onto the barbicel next to it.

A feather looks like a firmly attached mesh, but you can part it easily between barbs. Then, if you run your fingers over the feather, you can smooth it together so that you cannot tell where it was parted.

The feathers that you are most familiar with are called *contour feathers,* because they give the bird's body its contour, or shape. (A plucked chicken has a very different shape from a live chicken with all its feathers.) Contour feathers are used for warmth, and also to provide surfaces for the air to push against during flight. They usually grow in patterns on the bird's body. If you part a bird's feathers, you will discover that many parts of its skin are actually bare.

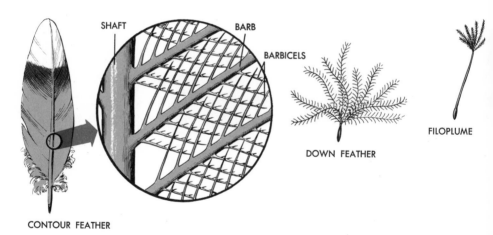

CONTOUR FEATHER SHAFT BARB BARBICELS DOWN FEATHER FILOPLUME

Kinds of feathers.

In addition to the contour feathers, birds have two other types. *Down feathers* are fluffy tufts that do not have a central shaft. Baby birds have only down feathers. In adult birds, the down feathers grow close to the body and are usually hidden by the contour feathers. They help to keep the bird warm. *Filoplumes* (FILL-uh-PLOOMZ) are a third type of feathers. Their name means "thread feathers," and they look like threads or hairs.

Like the hair of mammals, feathers are nonliving materials that are produced in living sheaths in the skin. It will hurt a bird if you pull one of its feathers out, but it will not hurt it to have its feathers cut. When ostrich feathers were in fashion, these big birds were raised by the millions on ostrich farms, and their feathers were clipped every eight months or so. Often birds lose their feathers, or molt, and grow new ones to replace them.

If you look closely at a bird, you will find that not all of its body is covered with feathers. Its legs are covered with small scales. A number of other animals have scales that help to protect them. Fish have horny scales that are covered with a slimy secretion. The scales of reptiles are quite dry. Parts of the dermis and the epidermis combine to make these scales, which are usually lapped over one another like the shingles on a roof. The scales are embedded in the skin, just as your fingernails are embedded in the skin of your fingers.

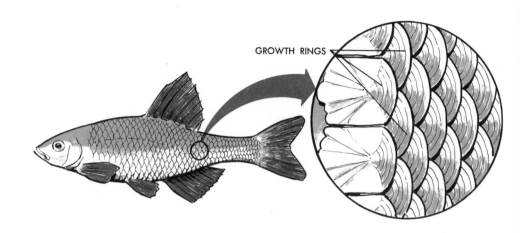

GROWTH RINGS

A fish's age can be told from its scales.

Did you know that you can tell how old a fish is by looking at its scales? A fish scale has growth rings, like the growth rings in the trunk of a tree. As a fish grows, its scales get larger by adding more horny material around the edges. In the summer, food is plentiful and the fish grows quickly. A broad, light-colored band forms around each of its scales. In the winter, food is scarce and the fish grows more slowly. The winter growth ring on its scales is narrow and dark. By counting the pairs of light and dark rings on a fish scale, you can tell exactly how old it was when it was caught, and even what season of the year it was when it died.

The tips of your fingers and toes are protected by another horny, nonliving product of your skin.

The part of your nails that you can see is dead, but they grow out of living nail roots, hidden under a flap of skin at the base of the nail. The nail plate is made of thick, tough layers of flat cells. Keratin gives them their stiffness and strength. Are there any white spots or black-and-blue marks on your nails? You may notice that as weeks go by, these spots move down the nail bed until they finally reach the end of the nail and are cut or filed or broken away. These spots are usually marks of injury to the nail that occurred in the part that was still alive. If you make a small scratch in one of your nails, just above the cuticle, and measure how far down it has moved each week, you can see for yourself how fast nails grow. Fingernails grow about a tenth of a millimeter each day. (Hairs grow about three-and-a-half times as fast.) You can replace a whole fingernail in about three or four months.

What good are fingernails? Unless you cut or bite your nails very short, you probably find them helpful in picking up small items. Fingernails also help to protect the ends of the fingers from bruises and cuts. Toenails help to protect the ends of the toes.

Many animals have specialized nails that can be used for various things. Birds' nails are shaped into pointed claws, which help them to grasp a perch on a tree branch or clutch and tear their prey. Tree-climbing animals, from cats to koalas, usually have claws that can dig into the tree trunks. Lions use their claws to tear food apart.

Perhaps the strangest kind of "nail" is the horse's hoof. This thickened, toughened structure makes such an effective shoe that it seems astonishing to think that a horse actually runs about on a single modified toenail on each foot!

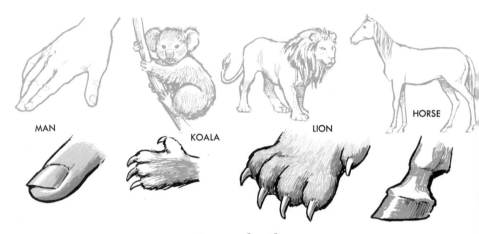

MAN

KOALA

LION

HORSE

Types of nails.

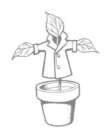

8
Plant "Skin"

Plants have many of the same problems as animals. Their delicate tissues must be protected from bruises and microbes, and they must be shielded from drying out. Most plants solve this problem by producing a waterproof "overcoat" that covers their leaves and stems.

The plant's epidermis is made up of a single layer of cells, which fit together like a jigsaw puzzle. The waterproofing is supplied by a waxy film, called the cuticle, which covers the epidermis.

You might guess that the green color of plant leaves and stems comes from a pigment in the epidermis. If you did, you would be only half-right. The green color is produced by a green pigment, *chlorophyll* (KLORE-OH-FILL). But the chlorophyll is found in the deeper tissues of the plant, under the epidermis. The epidermis is so thin that you can see the green color through it. Light rays can pass in through the plant's epidermis, and their energy is used by the plants to make food materials.

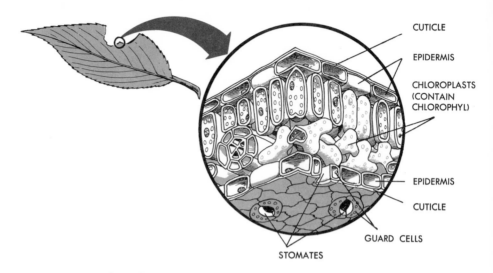

CUTICLE

EPIDERMIS

CHLOROPLASTS
(CONTAIN
CHLOROPHYL)

EPIDERMIS

CUTICLE

GUARD CELLS

STOMATES

Plant leaves are covered by epidermis, too.

This process is called *photosynthesis* (FOE-TOE-SIN-THE-SISS).

Plants need certain raw materials for photosynthesis. They need water, which they get from the ground through their roots. They need carbon dioxide, which is a gas found in the air. But carbon dioxide cannot pass through the waxy cuticle that covers the plant leaves and stems. This gas gets into the plants through tiny openings in the leaves. These openings are called *stomates* (STOH-MATES), and they are like gates that can be opened or shut. Each stomate is guarded by two special epidermal cells, shaped like tiny kidney beans. These cells are called *guard cells,* and they are unusual in several ways.

78

First of all, the guard cells are green. They are the only epidermal cells that contain chlorophyll. They have the ability to change their size. When the guard cells swell up, they close the stomates. When they shrink, they open them.

During the day, when the sun is shining brightly, the stomates are wide open. Gases can pass freely in and out of the leaves. But the plant pays a price for its supply of carbon dioxide. It loses a great deal of water through its open stomates. Since it needs water for its chemical reactions and to help hold its cells firm and stiff, the plant must take in enormous amounts of water through its roots all the time.

The stomates help the plant to save water. During the night, when no sunlight energy can reach its chlorophyll, the plant does not need carbon dioxide for photosynthesis. And so its guard cells swell, and its stomates are nearly closed.

Plant roots are covered by an epidermis, too, but they do not have a waxy cuticle. If they did, they would be waterproof, and then they would not be able to take in water from the soil. Water passes freely through the thin, delicate epidermis of the tiny root hairs.

Have you ever tried to dig a hole in the soil with your hand? There are many sharp, rocky particles that can scratch and hurt you. This is exactly what

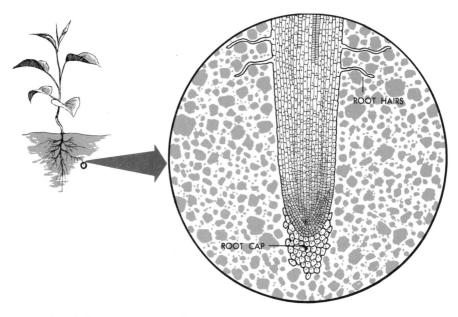

ROOT HAIRS

ROOT CAP

The delicate root epidermis is protected by a cap on the tip.

would happen to plant roots if they tried to push their way through the soil with only a delicate epidermis to cover them. Yet they do push their way through the soils as they grow. The growing tips of plant roots are protected by a thimble-shaped cap of tough cells called a *root cap*. As the root tip pushes its way through the soil, the outer cells of the root cap are continually worn away and replaced by new ones that are formed by the root epidermis.

Some plants have soft green stems, which are covered by the same kind of epidermis as the leaves. But others have woody stems, which are covered by bark. The bark of trees and bushes contains a layer of cork, which is formed just under the epidermis of the stem. Gradually, a fatty or waxy substance seeps into the outer cork cells. After a while, the epidermis is cut off from its supply of food and water, and so it dies and scales away.

The cork of tree bark is a good protective covering. It cuts down the loss of water from the stem and protects the tree from invading fungi and other microbes. It is an insulating blanket that protects the stem from cold, and it may even protect the living tissues of the tree from fires.

Did you know that when you eat the skin of a baked potato, you are eating cork, like the cork in tree bark? When a potato tuber is first formed, it is covered by a very thin layer of cork that can easily be scraped off. But after it has been stored for a while, the cork layer gets thicker and helps to protect the potato tuber from rotting.

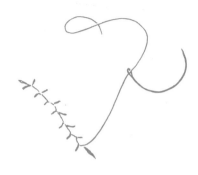

9

Frontiers of Skin Research

Do you have any scars on your skin? Perhaps you fell down the stairs when you were smaller, and had to get stitches in your head. Perhaps you had a bad cut or burn. Some people have such bad scars that they cannot move their fingers or some other part of the body properly. Or they may have scars that distort the features of the face and make them seem ugly. This can make a person very unhappy and can change his whole life.

Doctors have been researching for many years for ways to help people with problems like these. One of the techniques they use is *skin grafting*. A piece of skin is transplanted from another part of the body. Eventually it grows in its new place as though it had been there all the time. But until a new blood supply has been established, part of the skin that is being removed must be left attached to its old place on the body. Afterward it is cut off, and new skin grows over the spot from which it was taken.

Skin grafting takes advantage of the skin's amazing ability to repair itself. But it is often a very difficult process, and the patient must spend weeks or months with one part of his body uncomfortably attached to another. Surgeons are trying to find better ways to help the skin to help itself.

They have found, for example, that if a large area of the body is burned, new normal skin cannot cover the whole area by itself. Many skin grafts would be needed to cover it. But if the grafted skin is cut up into a criss-crossed lattice and laid over the whole burned area, the open spaces will gradually fill up with new skin. After a year or two, the whole grafted area may heal without scars or signs of the unusual skin graft that was made.

Doctors are also working on artificial materials that could be placed on damaged skin to stimulate the growth of new skin. A mesh of fibers made from the protein *collagen* (KOLL-a-jen), which is a part of normal skin, has been tried. Researchers are also experimenting on the use of an enzyme,

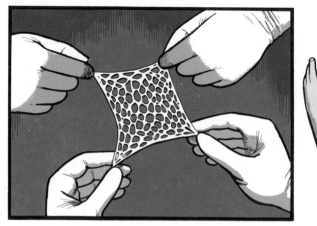
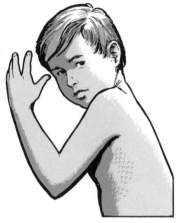

A new skin grafting technique. New skin will fill in the gaps, and the mesh pattern will disappear in about a year.

collagenase (KOLL-LAJ-EN-ASE), to dissolve out the collagen fibers in scar tissue. They hope that this will permit new, normal skin cells to fill in the gap.

Do you know what to do when you burn yourself? You may think that you should smear butter or some greasy salve on the burn. But doctors now think that this is not the best thing to do at all. Instead, you should soak the burned skin immediately in cold water. You will find that this treatment helps to stop the pain and makes the burn heal much faster.

Of course, a bad burn should be treated as soon as possible by a doctor. For a really bad burn, in which many layers of skin cells have been seared off, and the rest are charred and blackened, a surgeon may have to remove the damaged tissues so that the skin can heal. Patients with burns over large areas of skin are very hard to care for. They are very susceptible to infections, and they lose a great deal of moisture from their bodies. Medical researchers are working on many new techniques to help burn victims recover and to keep them more comfortable. They are even trying a new kind of hospital bed that suspends the burn patient on a cushion of air, so that his body does not touch the bedclothes.

Index